Table of Contents

Autism and Addiction: Exploring Substance Misuse in Autistic Individuals

1. Introduction to Autism and Addiction

1.1. Defining Autism Spectrum Disorder (ASD)

1.2. Understanding Addiction and Substance Misuse

2. Prevalence and Risk Factors

2.1. Prevalence of Substance Misuse in Autistic Individuals

2.2. Risk Factors for Developing Substance Misuse in Autism

3. Challenges in Diagnosis and Treatment

3.1. Diagnostic Challenges in Identifying Substance Misuse in Autistic Individuals

3.2. Unique Treatment Considerations for Autistic Individuals with Substance Misuse

4. Neurobiological and Behavioral Mechanisms

4.1. Neurobiological Underpinnings of Autism and Addiction

4.2. Behavioral Patterns and Characteristics in Autistic Individuals with Substance Misuse

5. Social and Environmental Factors

5.1. Impact of Social Skills and Social Isolation on Substance Misuse in Autism

5.2. Environmental Triggers and Protective Factors

6. Intervention Strategies and Best Practices

6.1. Behavioral Interventions for Substance Misuse in Autistic Individuals

6.2. Pharmacological Approaches and Considerations

7. Family and Caregiver Support

7.1. Role of Family and Caregivers in Supporting Autistic Individuals with Substance Misuse

7.2. Accessing Support Services and Resources

8. Ethical and Legal Considerations

8.1. Ethical Issues in Research and Treatment of Autism and Addiction

8.2. Legal Rights and Protections for Autistic Individuals with Substance Misuse

9. Future Directions in Research and Practice

9.1. Emerging Trends in Understanding Autism and Addiction

9.2. Innovative Approaches in Prevention and Intervention

Understanding the Relationship Between Autism and Substance Misuse

1. Introduction to Autism and Substance Misuse

2. Prevalence of Substance Misuse Among Autistic Individuals

3. Factors Contributing to Substance Misuse in Autistic Individuals

3.1. Sensory Sensitivities and Coping Mechanisms

3.2. Social Challenges and Peer Influence

3.3. Anxiety and Depression

3.4. Executive Functioning Difficulties

4. Protective Factors and Resilience in Autistic Individuals

5. Intersectionality: Gender, Race, and Socioeconomic Status

6. Challenges in Diagnosing Substance Misuse in Autistic Individuals

7. Impact of Substance Misuse on Autistic Individuals

7.1. Physical Health

7.2. Mental Health

7.3. Social and Occupational Functioning

8. Interventions and Treatment Strategies

8.1. Behavioral Therapies

8.2. Pharmacological Interventions

8.3. Family and Community Support Programs

9. Future Directions in Research and Practice

Autism and Addiction: Exploring Substance Misuse in Autistic Individuals

1. Introduction to Autism and Addiction

Attention deficit hyperactivity disorder (ADHD), a diagnosis characterized by symptoms of inattentiveness and/or hyperactivity, is a common co-occurring condition with ASD. The link between ADHD, ASD, and substance use has been studied; however, the links between these similar traits and substance abuse are still poorly understood. This essay will: 1. briefly explain the overlapping cognitive and emotional difficulties for ASD and substance disorders, focusing particularly on internalizing behaviors, emotion regulation, social interpretation, and empathy; and 2. explore the extent of substance misuse in those diagnosed with ASD. There is a paucity of empirical research into this under-investigated area in autism research; therefore, emphasis is placed on broader studies of personal strengths and vulnerabilities associated with ASD in order to hypothesize about the increasing likelihood of developing a substance and/or alcohol addiction. The use of broader autism studies in this essay provides an explanation for ASD younger individuals and adults, who may develop a relationship with drinking and drugs in hopes of acquiring these social connections in intoxication.

ASD refers to a group of presumed lifelong, multifaceted neurodevelopmental conditions. Autism Spectrum Disorder (ASD) and addiction are challenging, potentially debilitating, and often comorbid issues. There are many complex and interlinked reasons for this, ranging from accumulating life stresses to impairments in cognitive, social, and emotional functioning. Those with autism are often dealing with a flux of change, inside and out, that they don't understand or are able to control. Consequently, a significant manifestation of this can be found in issues of alcohol or controlled drug consumption. Substance misuse is, unfortunately, a significant problem in people affected with ASD. To further understand the impact of substance misuse on autistic individuals, a brief explanation of the co-occurring conditions of ASD and addiction is provided.

1.1. Defining Autism Spectrum Disorder (ASD)

Social areas of potential difficulty include communication, empathy, moral judgement, theory of mind, emotion recognition, eye contact, face processing, and people seeing autistics as being "weird" due to social interaction impairments. Autistic individuals sometimes experience an ongoing feeling of social failure, barriers to friendship, and rejection and are at elevated risk for panic disorder, depression, female sex of birth, and mental health issues. These problems could be exacerbated by a diagnosis of autism. For example, suggest that adult autistic women experience elevated rates of bipolar and anxiety disorders as opposed to their male counterparts. Additionally, this group had a higher prevalence of bipolar disorder than their counterparts in the local population. Autistic individuals sometimes take drugs to self-medicate autistic symptoms of stress and poor sleep quality, as well as impaired mental health, suggesting that drugs of abuse could be reparative for the damaged brain. Regular use of illegal drugs in an attempt to relieve social angst—stated by a famous autistic woman—indicates that it may be more prevalent than observed and self-medication.

Autism Spectrum Disorder (ASD) is characterised by abnormalities in two fundamental psychological processes: social interaction and communication, alongside restricted and repetitive interests and activities. Core features associated with ASD include the ability to feel empathy, understand another person's perspective, share affect, and respond to social and emotional cues for the sole purpose of forming and maintaining relationships. Deficits in social cognition, the means by which one computes and organises information about people and social situations to reflect behaviour, moral reasoning, and critical reasoning, coupled with a desire for social acceptance and inclusion, can give rise to a potentially potent risk factor for drug experimentation in both boys and girls: peer pressure.

1.2. Understanding Addiction and Substance Misuse

The current understanding of addiction and substance misuse involves the psychological and biological underpinnings of the disorder. Simply put, an addiction disorder can be understood as a dysfunctional neuro-cognitive processing of both reward and punishment cues, where reward systems are attributed exaggerated salience and punishment systems toward all forms of drug-related stimuli are blunted. Addicts persistently feel the urge to recreate the effects of the addictive substance. Post-mortem studies on drug addicts have shown brain atrophy and dysregulation in the transmission of messages, which are suggestive of changes in the brain. Withdrawal can and does present as a deterrent of its own, with symptoms such as insomnia, nausea, anxiety, irritability, and low moods, all of which prompt further use of drugs to overcome them.

Many of us have had a friend, family member, or colleague who struggles with addiction. With 223.3 million people worldwide reporting substance misuse and 36.3 million people meeting criteria for dependence on substances, more than ever, addiction and substance misuse have become progressive problems shining through the ambient noise. Although there are multiple discourses about how to identify what addiction really is, most modern definitions include it being a chronic, relapsing disorder which is characterized by compulsion (and obsession), persistent use of drugs despite adverse effects, loss of control in limiting intake, and the emergence of a negative emotional state when access to the substance is removed. In essence, two kinds of addiction exist: behavioral and substance.

2. Prevalence and Risk Factors

In order to begin this process, it is important to more fully understand the overall prevalence of substance misuse among autistic individuals. Unfortunately, a definitive conclusion on the association between autism and substance misuse is prevented by a great deal of variability within the literature. In an effort to compensate for the variability in prevalence across the literature, we can also employ comparisons with non-autistic control individuals. Prevalence estimates for substance misuse in autism can range from 3% of 10 individuals to 60% of 55 individuals. Such wide discrepancies in prevalence between different studies are likely reflective of differing sample sizes and demographic characteristics. However, the population-based prevalence of alcohol and substance misuse ranges from 7.4% among 44,825 individuals to 12.6% in 2,126 individuals.

Substance use and misuse is a major public health concern. Current estimates indicate that 5.4% of the global population have suffered a substance abuse disorder over the last year. Substance misuse and addiction have traditionally been considered to be less common in autistic individuals due to an aversion to the sensation of being intoxicated. However, more recent research indicates a high rate of co-occurrence between autism and addiction. This highlights the need to more fully understand the relationship between autism and substance misuse.

2.1. Prevalence of Substance Misuse in Autistic Individuals

It is important to note that rates of substance misuse in autism do change based on an individual's intellectual level. For example, those with profound learning disability are at a much higher risk of developing substance misuse disorders than those who are typically of at least average intelligence.

In the general population, rates of substance misuse are around two to five percent. However, within the autistic population, studies have reported rates of anywhere from sixteen percent to almost fifty percent. The reality is likely to be somewhere in between because many autistic individuals in both studies never consumed alcohol at all.

In response, the recent existence of an international research project has been examining substance misuse in high-functioning autistic adults. This research is the first time that substance misuse in autistic individuals has been examined using a variety of methodologies to determine the true extent of this problem. As of this writing, data are still being collected. However, the preliminary results are extremely interesting and showcase the significant impact substance misuse has within the autistic community.

Recent research has established that rates of comorbid psychiatric conditions are high in autistic individuals. Anxiety, depression, and sleep disorders are all much more common in adults with autism when compared to the general population. Substance misuse, also referred to as addiction, is one such psychiatric presentation that has long been neglected in the literature.

2.2. Risk Factors for Developing Substance Misuse in Autism

Low intelligence, problems with communication and increased sensory sensitivities have also been suggested as potential risk factors for why someone with an ASD might misuse drugs. Each of these factors may make a person with autism more vulnerable to drug or alcohol misuse. Behavioral problems can have a considerable effect on child development and functioning. This can cause problems in the ability of people with autism to socialize and behave appropriately in a range of environments. Indeed, forming positive social networks with peers, being involved in a romantic-like relationship, and having a more positive perception of friendship are all factors that can reduce the risk of people with autism developing drug and/or alcohol addiction.

There are various risk factors associated with substance misuse. The first risk factor highlighted is another psychiatric diagnosis. There are a number of potential explanations about why people with autism may use drugs. For example, it may be that they are using the drugs as a form of self-medication to help them. They are also more likely to misuse substances if they have experienced abuse and bullying. This may include things such as emotional bullying, physical bullying or inappropriate online interactions with others. This may help to explain why people with non-autistic learning disabilities misuse drugs more than people with autism.

3. Challenges in Diagnosis and Treatment

The comorbid association between autism and substance misuse represents a clinical challenge for the identification and treatment of these occurrences. For clinical assessment, it is essential that the clinician is aware of the importance to identify both genuine cases of substance misuse and instances of hyperfocus on interests intrinsic to autism. Moreover, the often poor agreement between clinical assessment and biological screening suggests that a screening, with value-free results in false positive cases, is also advisable. Identification of substance misuse should be promptly followed by qualified intervention, particularly when external support constitutes one of the motivating factors. In fact, in autistic individuals with substance misuse, lack of motivation has been defined as an obstacle to the therapeutic process.

The situation is further compounded by the fact that it is difficult to define a precise boundary between substance misuse and addiction. The former refers to any patterns of use that could become maladaptive. However, from a psychological standpoint, the distinction between the two categories is not easy to define, especially because the consequences of non-severe substance misuse have often been overlooked. Another limiting factor is probably connected to difficulties in identifying the presence of a psychiatric disorder in individuals with ASC, particularly in those with intellectual, verbal, or cognitive impairment.

Many of the symptoms typically associated with substance misuse may be mistaken for autistic traits. Shared features, such as social difficulties, anxiety, unusual interests, and sensory sensitivities, may also blur the diagnostic focus.

3.1. Diagnostic Challenges in Identifying Substance Misuse in Autistic Individuals

Diagnostic challenges in identifying substance misuse in autistic individuals: idiosyncratic symptoms, such as anxiety, aggression, or self-stimulatory behavior, can be interpreted as symptoms of autism, whereas they might, in fact, be symptoms of an underlying substance use disorder. Substance misuse in the form of self-medication is more difficult to distinguish from other forms of substance use. Defining substance use as problematic in autism can be difficult, as some behaviors related to substance misuse align with the diagnostic criteria for autism, such as restricted and repetitive patterns of behavior and interests. In this instance, it is, of course, always important to remember that an individual may have a substance misuse disorder in addition to a diagnosis of autism. If there is a shift in the individual's functioning, treatment may be necessary; however, instances of substance-related shifts in functioning could conflict with the DSM-V criteria for autism and mislead reviewers. Some were some of the first to suggest that substance misuse in adults with autism may go undetected because the symptoms of abuse, as defined in the DSM-V, are also characteristics of autism. As a result, substance misuse may not be discovered unless a specialized assessment determines this to be the case. This will be an important area of future development in accelerating and expanding identification. In other work, some have suggested that changes in an individual's

Autism Spectrum Quotient could indicate substance misuse, but evidence for this remains inconclusive.

3.2. Unique Treatment Considerations for Autistic Individuals with Substance Misuse

Whether the diagnostic overshadowing and diagnostic overshadowing is explained by the inception of autism or by the simultaneous creation of autism and intelligence only in the view of the proto-"gods" in the 1940s researchers, it is manifest. Uninformed researchers observe that autism is primarily a cisgender, heteronormative male phenomenon that occurs in a specialized development of all the canonical information network with the exclusion of simulated processes.

The aim of this section is to discuss alternate speculative models of addiction in autistic individuals and the various intersections and comorbid links between unique behavioral and neurobiological factors in autism and substance misuse. This section speculatively proposes that there is no single best ideal treatment or etiological model of addiction that suits or applies to all autistic people, in part because of the unique ways in which addiction might arise in autism. Thus, further research is warranted.

This section will discuss the unique challenges in substance misuse for autistic individuals, with a focus on the theoretical proposition of mind-blindness and interoceptive processing, therapeutic interventions, and the experiences of people who have lived with dual diagnoses.

In clinical settings, there are numerous challenges in managing addiction within the context of autistic individuals. Behavioral addictions, which do not rely on the consumption of substances, can be particularly challenging for autistic individuals, and a higher co-occurrence of autism has been reported among individuals receiving treatment for substance misuse. Research has also shown a link between sensory issues and pain sensitivity in autistic individuals. This, coupled with emotional and cognitive distress, means that autistic individuals should be less likely to initially start using substances, formally speaking.

4. Neurobiological and Behavioral Mechanisms

There is a growing body of evidence associating autism and addiction, though little empirical work exists examining neurobiological or theoretical reasons for this association. For those studies that do exist, general characteristics of drug-using autistic individuals are suggested to involve adherence to the drug as a rigid way of avoiding novelty, normative social interaction, and overwhelming sensory inputs. Early findings conclude that results cannot necessarily be generalized to all drug-addicted autistics, and that amassing further data will be necessary before drawing stronger conclusions. A case report from describes a 30-year-old man with Asperger's who recovered from alcohol-use disorder and was at lower risk for addiction to multiple drugs because of adherence and OCPD. described two cases of drug misuse by males with Autism Spectrum Disorder. While studies examining the neurobiological similarities between autism and addiction are preliminary at this time, they represent an important next step in furthering our understanding for at-risk or addicted autistics.

As described in the prior section, both autism and addiction are associated with atypicalities in brain regions involved in social processing. Such areas include, but are not limited to, the frontal and cingulate cortices, striatum, amygdala, and mirror neuron system. Importantly, the rewarding effects of acute drug use typically include increases in social functioning and associated social brain regions. Chronic use is generally associated with a neuroadapted social system, or the reluctance to continue drug use in a social context, despite continued drug use without social presence. While the corresponding neurological atypicalities are not often discussed in relation to addiction research, decreased engagement with social brain regions is considered a core characteristic of autism. When measuring oxytocinergic responsivity during monetary exchange with a friend or stranger, reduced hypothalamic activation is observed in response to partner-versed friends but not strangers in autism. It has been posited that addiction shifts behavior to a socially-isolated model of drug use.

A growing body of literature points to two cardinal tiered neurobiological issues that may lead to the neurobiology of autism: first, issues that exist on the especially macro hole filled in by a patient's serotonin secretion and, second, the effect of oxytocin in autistic cognition, two neurobiological effects which have also been directly linked to addiction biology. The results of behavioral investigations and neuroimaging investigations show that people with ASD have showing a particular need for oxytocin, such people suggest anthropophobic behavior, as well as affective intuition, like lower levels of tolerance to alter and levels of fear as infants obtained in their ordained treatments. Autistic patients, therefore, have a missing hormone level, which can increase the incentive to medicines. The benefits of oxytocin treatment in having better interpersonal skills and in reducing repetitive actions and mannerisms have been confirmed. Aside from having autistic characteristics, many genes directly linked to ASD also play a direct technological part in the initiation and course of medicine dependence, covering genes linked to the ion channels, to important neurotransmitter secretion, and to the making of synaptic proteins. Moreover between people with ASD and as they age, serotonin seems to have a big neurochemical performance, and the flatten of the hormone can have a consequence on infralimiting interest in drugs because one psychiatric learning has thoroughly exposed that the more low insertion of serotonin in the body was the less concerned the individuals if they drank alcohol.

Fundamental neurobiological issues provide a useful perspective for articulating the potential comorbid psychopathologies between autism and substance abuse. Given the complicated symptomatology of autism, pinpointing precise neurological underpinnings that drive autistic behaviors can be a very challenging endeavor. Interestingly, however, there is a growing literature that perfectly illustrates the neurobiological connections between autism and comorbid schizophrenia, distinguishing this comorbidity as "an area of apparent overlap" with autism. Among the most common of these comorbidities are schizophrenia, anxiety disorder, mood disorders, and attention-deficit hyperactivity disorder, to name a few; comorbid diagnoses of each are associated with a higher risk of substance abuse.

4.2. Behavioral Patterns and Characteristics in Autistic Individuals with Substance Misuse

Frequency of use: The behavioral patterns clearly indicate dependency and considerable substance misuse over a long period of time. These specific patterns of use tend to point towards polydrug use and above-average levels of daily usage. Service use and high-risk behaviors indicate dual diagnosis (which means a mixture of autism and mental health problems). It is very likely that autistic individuals would need more help than the average substance abuser or dependent person due to behavior problems. Ethical considerations must also be taken into account, including the need to adapt interventions such as mutual aid groups. In the future, a qualitative study potentially informed by autistic individuals' experiences might serve to indicate how the doctor/therapist can assist in removing the considerable stigma these clients face, raising the chances of early interventions.

One of the key characteristics of autistic individuals is the presence of challenging behavior. These are behavior patterns that are difficult or different. Our participants reported problems with taking medication. This refers to an unwillingness to obey and also indicates a high prevalence of involuntary hospital admissions. The key characteristics of autism are social and communicational impairments, a preference for routine and sameness, resistance to change, and a difficulty in processing sensory information. The behavioral impairments manifest themselves in a number of ways. While we can think that substance misuse in autistic individuals is linked with escape and relaxation, it may also be due to behaviors influenced by cognitive differences and emotional regulation.

5. Social and Environmental Factors

It should be noted, however, that various papers argue for a strong neuropathological and genetic influence on addiction in autism and, looking beyond autism, that couples-based and social network approaches may not always be appropriate or suitable in all addiction contexts. However, social and structural processes, including isolation, might mediate substance misuse or protect against addiction in certain unusual populations. In sum, the social learning perspectives outlined previously might conceptualize a mature network with drug-using models, seeing the autistic individuals in such networks as being relatively malleable and naive in their views, particularly if they have not previously used substances. Consequently, their drug-using peers may be influential, requiring educational programs to focus on the wider social networks of these autistics. The idea that autistic individuals might be unusually vulnerable to substance misuse due to their misunderstood intentions and apparent non-conformity should also be examined in greater depth, as it is consistent with earlier findings. Further qualitative research is warranted to further unravel these surprising and novel potential social influences on substance misuse in autism.

The social challenges and altered social perception that characterize autism may affect patterns of substance misuse. Reduced social skills are associated with substance misuse in autism, a finding that interacts with findings from non-autistic populations. Loneliness might drive misuse of substances with effects on social behavior. Aversive social experiences and perceived rejection could increase the risk for misuse of coping motives to "up-regulate" distressing experiences. Furthermore, the influence of social networks on use of alcohol might further impinge on patterns of alcohol misuse in autistics.

5.1. Impact of Social Skills and Social Isolation on Substance Misuse in Autism

Autistic individuals also often struggle with social skills and can tend to isolate themselves because they feel they are different from those around them and are unsure about how to act in social situations, thus adding to their feelings of social anxiety. Substance misuse can help autistic individuals to feel better in the short term, and they may feel more like they 'fit in' or share a common interest with others in order to make friends and not be isolated. An individual's personal experience of loneliness and social isolation has been found to be predictive of cannabis use. As these individuals then continue to use substances to help ease these 'uncomfortable' social settings, they are at a higher risk of developing a substance misuse problem.

Social skills are behaviors that allow a person to interact with other people in a positive way. When a person has difficulty in these areas, they may struggle to form and keep effective relationships, and may isolate themselves from other people. Social isolation due to a lack of social skills can lead to an increased chance of substance misuse because of the risk effect of not having people around to support in times of need. Research has suggested that both the development and continuation of substance misuse are linked to poor social skills. Negative peer relationships, social isolation, and an increased risk of victimization due to having a neurodevelopmental condition such as autism can all be contributing factors to developing maladaptive coping strategies such as substance use and misuse.

3. Escapism from sensory: In this increasingly competitive, digital world, young people are often worn down to what feels like a low at an early age. Even people who are comparably successful are subject to explosive amounts of cortisol, and not everyone has the inner resources or external resources to cope with the effects of early signs of burnout. Help is subjective and skin in the eye of the beholder and cannot be solved with a cookie cutter one-size-fits-all approach.

2. Lack of social integration: A lack of friendships and an excess of promiscuous bullying lead to a sense of isolation and a lack of social supports—hardships known to be associated with both a diagnosis of autism and subsequent poor mental health by virtue of lacking this protective buffer. Importantly, low self-esteem and lack of sensation are proposed to play a bigger role in self-medication than autism or trauma.

1. Intersectionality: The identity of a person who struggled with sensory and emotional processing is considered to be fundamentally different from people with PTSD, suggesting difficult experiences of stigma within traditional treatment services. Indeed, two control groups, autistic people with comorbid PTSD and non-autistic prisoners, are found to have lower rates of self-reported substance use (54), which supports the notion of substance use being more strongly demarcated from normativity by intersecting factors in autism beyond the presence of inherent personality traits.

It has been suggested by people on the autism spectrum, parents, and professionals that seeking to understand the biopsychosocial context of self-medicating in autism could extend current thinking around addiction in this community. Key themes emerging from preliminary qualitative work (detailed in the above section 5.1.1) which center on why the environment might trigger substance use are as follows:

6. Intervention Strategies and Best Practices

Scientists are considering the use of treatments such as naltrexone, acamprosate, and the opiate antagonist nalmefene within clinical trials and within standard care for alcohol misuse and abuse. In this section, further issues faced by the clinician when working with this group of individuals are discussed. First, strategies for intervention need to be tailored towards this population. Research at present is limited with no large-scale papers available with randomized control trials. This is an area that can be worked upon, with surgeons and physicians actively discussing the need for research in this area.

Several face-to-face intervention strategies for individuals with autism who misuse substances have been described in the clinical literature. Some individuals have utilized the principles of cognitive behavioral therapy (CBT) to develop novel interventions tailored to the unique processing style often utilized by individuals with ASD. Using this type of approach, the individual needs of the person with autism can be taken into account and the therapy adapted according to these needs, for example using a more structured and concrete approach to therapy. For those individuals with autism who misuse alcohol, an emphasis on visual supports may have added value. Using visual information which is inherently less complex than verbal language and always present within the environment may ensure maximum comprehension and therefore there is the potential for visual aids to be helpful in reducing the misuse of alcohol and promoting positive mental and physical health. Pharmacological treatments have also been utilized in this population.

6.1. Behavioral Interventions for Substance Misuse in Autistic Individuals

The offers spectrum-specific directions to stimulate your thinking, give counsel and ideas whether you are a seasoned professional currently working with or one who may in the future work with individuals and families in this situation, or if you are a parent, carer, or person interested for a variety reasons in the ASD (perhaps Asperger) world. Part of the clinical management of adults diagnosed with alcohol dependence includes screening for autism. Cue, demands widening the knowledge base of the links between the two to include differing research paradigms and conditions.

In presenting these issues, we aim to inspire and stimulate the development and evaluation of interventions designed with the specific needs of an autistic substance-misusing population. Many, perhaps all, of the suggestions offered in the following paragraphs have borne their fruit in the field of neurotypical substance misuse; thus they carry with them the same risks and potential. Some of these suggestions may require minor variation between autistic populations defined by gender, age, functioning IQ, and other reasons, as they do in exploring autistic factors that may impact on treatment engagement in general fully or in part, and by targeting strategies at those alcohol-dependent clients in the context of an average mental age.

This section offers recommendations for behavioral intervention components specifically designed to aid autistic individuals who misuse substances. It is not intended to offer a definitive description of the clinical management of substance misuse in this population, as the current state of evidence for pharmacological, behavioral, and combined approaches is yet to offer a precise presentation of an appropriate management package, although some promising results are evident.

The demands of autism and addiction render a comprehensive understanding of one population invaluable to professionals working with the other. Offering tailored behavioral interventions to assist autistic individuals who struggle with substance misuse requires this level of specificity. This interaction between autism, personality, and comorbid conditions offers yet more evidence of the benefits of translating insight from one population to another.

6.2. Pharmacological Approaches and Considerations

In a targeted study of adults in the UK, OUD was found to be a significant concern in one clinical sample of autistic adults when compared with the general population. Despite this, whilst evidence for targeted medication supports its use in the general population, caution would suggest that a distinct and cautious approach should be taken not merely to treat disorder symptoms, but to also understand how new medications may interact with autism. There are four medications tested in the general adult population specifically treating OUD: methadone, buprenorphine, naltrexone, and naloxone. This indicates that these should be used selectively in the autistic population. Contrary to the use of pharmacotherapy in the general adult population, the literature seeks to understand not only the lack of any impact but the appropriateness in consideration of the developmental needs of the autistic child/adolescent. Any further guidelines to develop should possibly ensure not only best practice investigatory work for pharmacotherapy in addiction in children and young people, but also the essential process and outcomes desired in those with identified comorbid psychiatric conditions, particularly ASD/OUD.

Addressing co-occurring mental health conditions can help provide strong foundations for preventing or treating SUD/OUD. However, medication for comorbid psychopathologies may not directly reduce substance misuse per se in autistic individuals. Nonetheless, co-occurring mental health conditions, including those that directly influence risk for SUD/OUD, are a significant concern for many autistic individuals. Given high rates of co-occurring mental health conditions for autistic individuals facing addiction, particularly anxiety and depression, incorporating mental health care is an important consideration to managing substance misuse in this population. While this falls outside the bounds of this review, it is a consideration not to be ignored for future research.

7. Family and Caregiver Support

Autistic individuals are more likely to engage with both formal and informal supports if they involve family members. Indeed, families are frequently seen as natural supports by healthcare professionals. Research has established for some time that imposing guilt on family members for factors they believe they have some degree of control over (like an individual's substance misuse) can lead to family caregivers overextending themselves to be seen as performing "good" care. Family support can significantly aid compliance, especially if the autistic person is removed from their natural environment to the rigid structure of in-house, residential rehabilitation programs. This places unique responsibility on several interconnected layers of support networks or "systems" for people with more complex, dual-diagnoses and learning difficulties generally. Programs need to engage with the needs, priorities, and shared perspectives of these individuals to be successful. Ultimately, the aim of working with families and taking account of their perspectives on caring and "addiction" is to have a positive indirect and direct impact on the autistic individual in recovery.

The management of addiction for autistic individuals frequently relies heavily on significant others, such as immediate and extended family or caregivers (known as "families" and "family", respectively, from this point on). Families may often assume the primary role in helping someone to address their substance misuse and other self-injurious behaviors related to addiction, such as disordered eating, for example. It could be argued that family supports more people relative to the smaller number of in-house residential rehabilitation support programs, while also being involved yet further still through non-structured, non-residential mutual groups or "drop-ins" without longer-term profile.

7.1. Role of Family and Caregivers in Supporting Autistic Individuals with Substance Misuse

7.1. Role of Family and Caregivers in Supporting Autistic Individuals with Substance Misuse Family and caregivers play a very important role in supporting the individual with a dual diagnosis of being both autistic and having a substance misuse problem. Sometimes family members can give the best possible description of the autistic person and are more likely to admit involvement in the dual diagnosis. Being autistic has an impact on the lifestyle of the individual, especially in relation to the fact that the autistic may be more willingly open and honest, according to what their beliefs and how they see society. This means that it is much easier for the individual to admit to their drug or alcohol addiction, and once admitted to seek treatment. Caregivers need to be open, encouraging, understanding and supportive, and show respect for the choices of the family member or person they care for. Forming an alliance with the family will pave the way for itinerary to be agreed for the autistic individual, ensuring his or her full cooperation.

7.0. Family and Caregivers It is recognized that the family and caregivers are a crucial support system for the autistic individual who has the dual diagnosis of a substance misuse problem. Although substance misuse is often listed as one of the main stressors for carers of autistic adults, it is likely that the majority of support literature will be based on clinical experience of families or individual case studies. Therefore, their advice may overlook the vast variations in the complex needs of the autistic individuals with the dual diagnosis, as well as the varying levels of the problems caused. However, qualitative studies have been conducted with autistic individuals, family carers and professionals addressing some of the challenges that may be encountered by the individual, family and service providers.

Outline: 7.0. Family and Caregivers, 7.1. Role of Family and Caregivers in Supporting Autistic Individuals with Substance Misuse

7.2. Accessing Support Services and Resources

Family members of individuals showing symptoms of comorbid addiction show higher levels of stress and initiate more drug-related conversations in their attempts to assist in recovery efforts. The community mothers for at-risk teens Internet intervention. In the USA, the National Institute on Drug Abuse is the Federal agency that supports research on addiction and the development of evidence-based interventions to prevent and treat the disease. They have conducted and published research on the most effective ways to communicate with an addicted person so that they will agree to seek help. In order to aid American families in having such a conversation, federal funds for the community mothers intervention were used to build and maintain a website on addressing drug-related issues which contributed to the staff's ability to be recruited and retained in the trial.

Autistics can struggle to access services that are not adapted to their specific needs and which should take account of the impact of these adaptations on their service users' mental health. The family of an autistic person may also access the generic substance misuse service in the first instance, this is also known to happen in the United Kingdom for learning disabled individuals. Another support avenue for carers is to get help for themselves. The UK charity Al-Anon Family Groups supports anyone whose life is or has been affected by someone else's drinking. It is possible therefore for a friend or family member of an autistic person to get support for their own issues which arise from another's substance misuse.

There are a number of support services available for autistic individuals with a dual diagnosis of substance misuse. This includes specialist services targeted at autistic individuals, and generic substance misuse and addiction recovery provisions. At the most basic level, there is the generic substance misuse service aimed at the general population. This is usually the first point of contact for an individual in difficulty. Since the prevalence of autism is relatively low, and may not be the initial barrier to successful receipt of generic services, some autistics may miss out on specialist support because they are accessing generically orientated services.

8. Ethical and Legal Considerations

Individuals with autism and addictions are safeguarded from the health consequences of addiction through legislation that ensures equal access to health and support services. They are also covered by preventative legislation covering disability discrimination. For children, their behavior must be seen as neurodiverse and not criminal, ensuring rehabilitation is the focus of any juvenile justice system. When an individual with autism offends and is processed through the criminal justice system, they are able to access the full range of autism-specific services required. Individuals with autism and addictions are not processed differently in a legal system sense but should gain access to the mental health and advocate support they require as a result of criminal justice legislation.

The pool from which research and evidence for the treatment of addiction generally is drawn is a pool exclusively of those who have capacity, as determined by current metrics, policy, and legislation. There is, therefore, a dearth of research and clinical guidelines for the treatment of substance use disorders in those who are multiply marginalized in terms of capacity for decision-making processes. Moreover, autism is a profoundly under-researched area in the field of addiction. Therefore, standard treatments that are known to work for most people with SUDs might have different (worse) effects or not work in autism. Ethical concerns have been expressed about the validity of our understanding of the mechanisms underpinning the self-medication hypothesis and the subsequent delivery of well-established treatments without understanding the ways in which autism might interact with these processes. Outside of these concerns are the issues about knowledge and support for those individuals with both disabilities who go on to develop substance misuse problems. This includes support in accessing healthcare and the protections provided by legislation.

8.1. Ethical Issues in Research and Treatment of Autism and Addiction

Substance misuse is comparatively common in autistic individuals, yet research is limited and services currently fail to meet the needs of the dual diagnosis population. The practical implications of studying and addressing dual diagnosis result in a range of complex issues and concerns that must be addressed. Arguably, within this context, some of the major barriers are related to questions of capacity, consent, and power. Autism and addiction are widely misunderstood, stigmatized, and subject to negative societal perceptions. Questioning the extent to which it is legitimate to search for a disorder that is rarely studied invokes debates over causation and 'responsibility'. Autism research also raises broader bioethical concerns that touch on issues such as epigenetics and eugenics. Thus, stakeholders in this domain are motivated by a recognition that engagement in research might carry potential harms as well as opportunities for benefit. Indeed, negative attitudes in the general public and social exclusion of autistic people are known to be closely linked to the risk of developing associated mental health problems, including addiction. A central barrier to conducting integrated research for this population could therefore be viewed as a lack of awareness, or indeed quite possibly, cultural knowledge, regarding autism. For example, researchers in addiction may perceive autistic individuals as 'not a priority' or not representing 'existing services and client base'. In essence, the pivotal ethical dilemma is whether to even attempt to make the adaptation and innovation that is required, accept the diversity of the population, or whether the challenges and obstacles are viewed as insurmountable. Is a dual diagnosis research agenda a waste of time? Despite procedural ethical approval, can it be viewed as inherently 'wrong' to study this population of people?

8.2. Legal Rights and Protections for Autistic Individuals with Substance Misuse

Furthermore, the documentary has a focus on the legal context of autism in independent diverse adults with substance misuse problems. Autism has been recognized and defined in human rights jurisprudence as a need for care and protection, and is concerned with the concept of "silence and personal freedom." In the UK and elsewhere, there are relatively strong legislative frameworks specifically for adults with disabilities such as autism associated with substance misuse, where dual diagnosis is relatively common. Autistic outpatients who are able to explore their addiction can reject offers of support. Failure to plead the abuse of a large group of autistic persons may constitute discrimination, entitling them to remedies in law. It may be possible to increase the likelihood of success in this approach by gaining the intervention understanding of any meltdowns.

The neurodiversity clause ensures that autistic individuals are not denied access to substance misuse services available to the neurotypical population. In addition, there are also laws in place aimed at safeguarding the rights of neurodiverse individuals who may be subject to the criminal justice system, including those who misuse substances. Under the Autism (Northern Ireland) Act 2011, the accused (or a legal representative) has the right to request a statement of topic on appropriate support for autistic individuals, necessary interventions, how best to communicate with the individual, and how best to understand how the individual communicates with non-autistic people. In addition, in England and Wales, the Youth Justice Board has put in place a multi-agency framework for action to deal with young autistic people in the criminal justice system.

9. Future Directions in Research and Practice

• The apparent benefits to caretakers of further study and explanation of apparent high error rates in seeking to prevent substance misuse for people with autism in residential care, perhaps with possible explanations in terms of 'aversion learning' that are also involved in schizophrenia studies. In practice, interventions on the functional similarities might be 'nudge' or 'boost' interventions promoting Non-Drug Reinforcement. Alongside new information, research could yield substantial promise for prevention and help for people diagnosed with autism. This might include help in minimizing the control of addiction in autism on mental health treatment response, helping relevance of personal genetic risk profiles, policymakers and professionals in choosing appropriate treatments on the basis of differences in the epigenetic (including microenvironmental) changes caused by drug-induced changes in initial state in individuals, and the potential relevance of early life experience(s).

• A wider testing of whether a health behavior model concept for understanding and prevention can be finalized (individual capability, as well as motivation and enabling environmental factors). Specifically, this might include comments on what further factors (individual differences in sensory and social experiences, strengths of perseveration and D-receptor-mediated focus of attention) might be involved in autism to sustain addictive substance use against intentions to quit.

• Real-world studies of autistic individuals' substance misuse, crossover studies in mental health care, and the qualitative nature of the emotional and cognitive attraction of addictive substances for autistic people (with or without intellectual disability).

Autism and addiction are rapidly emerging themes in the schizophrenia literature. Many questions remain, but some research activity that could advance new prospects in the understanding of the relationship between autism and addiction concerns:

9. Future Directions in Research and Practice

9.1. Emerging Trends in Understanding Autism and Addiction

The purpose of this Special Issue of Brain Sciences on Autism and the co-occurring diagnosis of addiction emerged from conversations about the need for understanding and attention to dual diagnosis as the emerging trend in research on autism spectrum disorders (ASD) and developmental disabilities. It is becoming increasingly clear that this co-occurring condition is a very precise point in the continuum of autism and co-occurring mental health disorders. The quest for understanding this diagnosis requires an interdisciplinary approach, as well as an examination of related constructs. Adolescents and adults have always been living with the co-occurring condition of dual diagnosis because they were not "outgrowing" their autism spectrum disorder (ASD). Developmental perspectives can benefit from understanding this trend; children are also likely to grow into adults while still having ASD. While living with the VIS-ASD questionnaire was initiated and is co-led by autistic leaders because people diagnosed with autism are more likely to provide answers that center portraying the experiences and realities of individuals with autism (ASD) more accurately.

The conceptualization and understanding of dual diagnosis of autism and addiction is constantly shifting and growing clearer. This is important to understand then that all facets of autism and addiction must be explored, including the realm of substance misuse within autistic individuals. The latest step in expanding our knowledge and research of addiction and dual diagnosis of autism and substance misuse are explored within the section.

Section 9.1: Emerging Trends in Understanding Autism and Addiction

9.2. Innovative Approaches in Prevention and Intervention

Cutting-edge Interventions and Approaches: Genetic profile-based and neural profile-based personalized medicine, a focus that has many new investigators and a burgeoning symposium APA and CINP, and as such, it is an exciting novel approach in the field of addictions. CBT is the primary approach taken for the treatment of anxiety in autism, and as substance abuse can be a form of self-medication for anxiety, this may be an ideal approach to also prevent, or treat, substance abuse in autism. As of now there is only one study that evaluates the efficacy of generic-CBT in treating illicit substance abuse in adults with high-functioning autism, but there is hope for future randomized controlled trials using this approach as an intervention for comorbid addictions. Development-review.

As there is a dearth of research and scientific knowledge, this aim presents various innovative, cutting-edge approaches developed for prevention and/or intervention of autism and addiction comorbidity. In order to guarantee the quality of proposed approaches, we overlooked methodologically weak strategies developed by clinicians, and/or any non-peer-reviewed "pop-psych" approach. These techniques are not reflected here. Instead, strategies based on scientific evidence of change or showing promise based on current scientific knowledge of addiction, autism (spectrum as well as single "neuro"-types), and/or comorbidity breeds were selected. Many cautionary words are expressed because of the need of further examination to guarantee the efficacy and safety of these methods, particularly when autistic individuals are involved and in light of potentially ambiguous evidence surrounding other related issues.

Understanding the Relationship Between Autism and Substance Misuse

1. Introduction to Autism and Substance Misuse

This essay provides the scope and approach for a recently completed study on these issues and is divided into three sections. First, it offers an overview of the state of knowledge that exists in this area, summarizing existing evidence on the links between autism and substance misuse. The following section takes a closer look at the existing research literature on the connections between autism and substance misuse, focusing particularly on a description of the extent of the problem, the nature of interactions between those with autism and those without, the ways in which substance misuse among those with autism may negatively impact their social care, and possible ways for support and intervention. For the same reasons, the literature review also briefly summarizes a number of studies on reasons for substance use among people with autism, as well as some work that has sought to provide support or intervention in this area. In the final section, the essay explores the implications for those involved or interested in responding to this problem, offering a number of specific or structural challenges posed by the issue of co-occurring autism and substance misuse.

Autism and substance misuse are of continuing concern to professionals and policymakers in both the criminal justice and social care fields. Yet, despite the increasing awareness of the relationship that exists between the two, many learners and practitioners struggle to understand and respond effectively to this issue. Such complexities are likely to be reflected in the case studies and other questions associated with this essay.

2. Prevalence of Substance Misuse Among Autistic Individuals

A recent meta-analysis found the rate of substance misuse disorders in diagnostic-stage autism to be 6%, with the combined use of alcohol and tobacco most common. A recent clinical study of Canadian teenagers found that around 13% of young autistic people had used an illicit substance, compared with just over 3% of a non-autistic comparison group. Another study reported that autistic individuals were between 1.27 and 1.52 times more likely to misuse alcohol or illegal drugs than the general public. Substances can be consumed in many different ways. The most common route of administration of substances was via smoking, followed by taking substances orally. Other methods of consumption included drinking alcohol, using a hookah, or via inhalation. The most used substances in the last year were alcohol (80.6%, 168) and cannabis (53.4%, 111), followed by vapes (40.9%, 85), tobacco (21.7%, 45), and waterpipes (13.0%, 27).

Substance misuse is a major problem throughout society. Recent estimates have indicated that around 250 million people use illegal drugs globally and around 3.3 million young people aged 15-16 have used drugs in the last year. Alcohol use is widespread, with 2.0 billion drinkers recorded globally in 2016, and 50 million people estimated to have some sort of alcohol use disorder. Almost 17 million people worldwide are estimated to misuse opiates. It is an offence to use and supply illegal drugs in England

and Wales as governed by the Misuse of Drugs Act 1971 and related laws, of which the maximum penalty is 7 years in prison for class A drugs (e.g., crack cocaine and ketamine) or 5 years/14 years in prison for class B/C drugs. In 2016/2017, 938,207 adults and 104,608 young people were prosecuted for drug offences in the UK.

3. Factors Contributing to Substance Misuse in Autistic Individuals

5.3. Various Dimensions of the Substance Misuse-ASD Relationship - Summary. As such, for some individuals, avoiding the many people in their lives who are substance users (or recovering substance users) and managing to avoid ever trying substances will be enough to prevent progression to substance misuse. For some, explaining negative consequences over relaxation effects can act as a buffer. For some others, explanation in terms of addiction's fatal consequences might sap the necessary relief from hedonic responses.

From the contents of the present review, it is evident that a multitude of factors contribute to substance misuse in the autism spectrum. The various influences tend to interact differently in different autistic people, contributing to a variety of risk profiles which manifest differently in terms of adverse consequences such as onset of substance misuse, addiction severity and treatment needs. A cumulative process is likely at work, such that when barriers are overcome or compensatory strategies no longer function, that person will be more likely to begin substance misuse or have problems with it. Given the fact that the factors contributing to the problem are so multi-faceted and can differ between individuals, it is clear that similarly diverse approaches will be needed to address the situation.

3.1. Sensory Sensitivities and Coping Mechanisms

Substances can be used as a means by autistic adults to mask overloads to sensory sensitivity that they feel unable to cope with or manage and/or as a means to self-medicate to relieve feelings of anxiety among other reasons. Autistic adults who were more sensitive to sensory stimuli were more likely to use alcohol and/or drugs whose primary effect is to reduce arousal, to help cope with and manage sensory and emotional difficulties. Given that alcohol can be used to reduce feelings of anxiety and depression and can be reported to calm down emotions, it is necessary for research to determine who is at risk of substance misuse, the cause of distress, and the mechanisms in place to address such issues, such as coping responses. While substance misuse to manage and cope with sensory sensitivity is not proposed to be more prevalent beyond a certain point of sensory sensitivity, other factors could suggest the need for alternative approaches. It is for this reason that this paper focuses on the relationship between two factors; namely sensory sensitivities as measured by a self-report measure of sensory processing and individual coping responses.

3.1.2. Substance misuse as a coping mechanism

Sensory sensitivities are a well-documented feature of autism. Autistic individuals often experience difficulties with sensory processing resulting in under and/or over-responsiveness to sensory stimulation, which can lead to sensory overwhelm that can be experienced as uncomfortable or painful. Autistic adults may experience reduced tolerance to sensory stimulation particularly in environments that are highly stimulating, such as noise, bright lights, and strong smells. Sensory deprivation is also a possible issue. Autistic people have also reported higher levels of adverse thoughts, feelings, and behaviors induced by sensory under and over-sensitivity compared to non-autistic individuals.

3.1.1. Autism and sensory sensitivities

3.2. Social Challenges and Peer Influence

There is already a sound evidence base that details how neurodevelopmental disorders in general, and autism in particular, can lead to a series of social challenges. Across the age range, the peer group will be the primary source to let people know how they are doing in terms of developing a personal identity. These roles of peers and how they can, and do, influence behaviour and expectations are also a significant driver in the development of values and one's place in society, for good or bad. Hamner and McEvoy suggest that "Mental illness can increase the impact of new peer groups by enhancing the individual's sense of hopelessness." This acquisition of identity and values is made alongside the development of both trust, or appropriate avoidance of uncertain actions and perceived risk in social interactions in general and in relationships with drugs in particular.

Section 3.2. Social Challenges and Peer Influence. It is also suggested that autistic individuals, ideally through a two-way process of informed decision making, need to be given the opportunity to express their view of their own health needs planning. Importantly, the panel and key informants identified a deep lack of evidence for and a priority for new research into understanding the specific challenges and needs of autistic individuals who misuse substances in different ways. For research findings to be valid and practically useful, they must be fed directly into a process of change that may vary for different groups in terms of literacy and support needs and opportunities at a national, regional, local and individual levels.

3.3. Anxiety and Depression

The use of alcohol and drugs is far higher (75%) than the general population (13%) among people with mild to moderate learning disabilities. Far less research has been focused specifically on substance use or misuse among adults diagnosed with autism than children. General factors which have been found to be linked to an increased use of drugs or alcohol include social isolation and bullying, low self-esteem, high fear of crime, and previous abuse. All of these factors are well documented both in the wider learning disability and autism literature.

There is only limited evidence to suggest a link between anxiety and depression among autistic adults, which could lead to substance use. This may be because it is difficult to disentangle primary and secondary emotional challenges (i.e., anxiety or depression driving substance misuse). Although more research is needed to confirm, some evidence suggests that depression is a component of autism. Such blunt systematically presented information drives feelings of worthlessness and isolation, and substance use. Certainly, autistic adults use pro-recovery social identities in relation to their mental health challenges and how to address them. Issues such as identity, disability pride, and how the notion of 'recovery' is considered within the autism community certainly as possible for mental health difficulties, and not engaging with drugs/substances, could all influence any reported association between autism, anxiety, depression, and mental health.

3.4. Executive Functioning Difficulties

This section examines the relationship between ASD and substance misuse through a bio-psycho-social lens. It analyses the profiles of individuals and highlights the fact that substance misuse negatively impacts on several social points of intervention identified within the study. This study presents a proposed group intervention that was piloted in 2019, and the effectiveness of this to reduce ASD young people's drug use, utilizing Bayesian statistics techniques. Substance use mis-education needs to account for the unique information processing of individuals across the autism spectrum. People with an autism diagnosis outperform neurotypical controls on detail processing but are outperformed by those without an autism diagnosis on context recall and on integrating new information with existing knowledge. While this capacity to focus on detail is often described as a cognitive strength and is not yet fully understood, the dispersed or weak central coherence hypothesis suggests looking at details at the expense of the surrounding context or integration into prior relational structures to be a cognitive deficit of autism. This ability to process detailed information in isolation can inadvertently assist in the development of myopic addiction schemas. In other words, rather than passively attuned to cues of the environment, autism may leave the individual more able to construct a detailed and idiosyncratic world of their own that desired drugs or activities would be likely to fit into, therefore tempting the individual with an autism diagnosis to drug or activity of choice.

3.4. Executive Functioning Difficulties. The autism spectrum has been identified as a risk marker for a gamble at risk and the development of a range of addictions. The risk for a level of lifetime substance dependence, compulsive addiction to or abuse of other substances is 3 to 4 times higher in those who have an autism diagnosis. The AS group used substances to look less socially awkward or self-medicate coercive symptoms; no such motivation emerged in the comparison group. Our study results indicate that individuals with AS are likely to misuse substances as a result of situational or interpersonal use based on impaired social judgement and a long-term poor decision-making based on their impaired sense of identity. Dependent users also had less insight into their own condition and about the opportunity to change their known patterns than those who were not dependent.

4. Protective Factors and Resilience in Autistic Individuals

The high percentage of individuals who do not misuse substances should also be borne in mind. By focusing on the protective factors, strengths, strategies, and internal and external resources utilised by many to create positive self-identities, or to enhance and bolster the lives of members of the autism community, this report seeks to fill gaps. Our aim is to systematically examine the factors and opportunities that can and do foster resilience and positive outcomes for individuals. There is a paucity of recent investigation in this area, and summarising a single pathway for surmounting disadvantage is not easy, since this is liable to vary for each of these intersecting dimensions. Moreover, this perspective can prove useful for examining the lives of members of the autism community in greater detail and realistically than the predominant concentrations on risk factors. These protective factors may well combat potential problems, or impact on others' abilities to mitigate them and must form a part of our output.

The evidence summarised in the foregoing sections of this report suggests that the risk of substance misuse in autistic populations is greater than those in the wider neurotypical community. However, it is necessary to accentuate that substance misuse is not a universal part of the lived experience of all individuals with autism, nor is it a predetermined feature of the condition.

5. Intersectionality: Gender, Race, and Socioeconomic Status

It is possible that both race and SES, through issues such as discrimination and lack of mental health care, may also differently impact the rates of substance misuse among G.I.D and T.D. individuals. This has implications for this paper because linking one's race or SES to substance misuse and other destructive behaviors can be perceived as stigmatizing, and therefore, the expectations of participants of color and/or low SES may be counterproductive. This is especially important to consider when the focus is on a population that may have distinct needs that differ from typical White, middle-class males. There is diversity within autism. Perhaps most notably, males are more likely to receive a diagnosis of autism than females. Analogous to the 'extreme male brain' theory of autism, studies of the non-autistic population have shown that gender differences in attitudes to health generally can have a profound effect on the way men may misuse substances in comparison to women, and that being male is one risk factor of many for categorization as poor sex health-wise. If too, the 'extreme male brain' theory of autism applies to attitudes to health and services, then perhaps adult men who are diagnosed later with an autism spectrum condition could be more likely to misuse substances than women. We have noted some specific research on substance users with autism, which shows the potential effectiveness of gender comparison and identification of women at risk.

Because the experience of autism intersects with gender, race, and socioeconomic status, further similarities or differences might be found in the way in which different autistic groups use alcohol, tobacco, or drugs, as the relationship between autism and misuse of substances can be influenced by further intersectional factors like these. Women with high functioning autism use smoking and drugs for self-medication longer in life stress than those from the general non-autistic population. Another study also reveals women with Asperger syndrome start smoking at a later age, suggesting there may be sex differences in the age at start of substance misuse between autistic and non-autistic women.

6. Challenges in Diagnosing Substance Misuse in Autistic Individuals

There is no direct way to diagnose substance misuse on the basis of clinical presentation and autistic individuals may be motivated to use both illicit and licensed substances by affective symptoms for which they have learned one of the few relief methods demonstrated to them. Polypharmacy is, therefore, common as some additional substance is suggested, added, or substituted as their confidence or funds vary. Autistic individuals may also be compelled by a desire for concreteness (which an illicit substance dealer will typically provide—working along the lines of social frames which they may or may not apply the term 'psychopath') or may be compelled to comply with grooming behaviors (once again, pop culture will hold up drug dealing as the epitome of adult behaviors).

A recent publication has proposed the development of tailored interventions for autistic adults at risk of substance misuse based on individual-level biological information and using current theories on substance misuse. This would be the first step in intervening with individuals whose autism has not yet been diagnosed as BSD patients are rarely diagnosed with autism. Unfortunately, current systems are not equipped to always recognize or diagnose autism nor to diagnose by reframing the behavior as substance misuse. Therefore, the first step will be to attempt to develop a system for early warning and referral which could be based on average group data in the literature. To use group data as predictors of individual behavior is always problematic.

7. Impact of Substance Misuse on Autistic Individuals

In the mental health continuum of individuals with autism, substance misuse's effects are complex and are also subject to varying reactions depending on the individual. Of concern is research by the NSPCC that reports rates of inadequate support which contribute to extant issues, including illicit drug use among individuals in contemporary society. By tackling the impact of substance misuse on individuals with autism, support can potentially have a concomitant effect. In addition to helping people lead a controlled lifestyle regarding their substance use, the effects include assisting in securing employment, training and meaningful activities. Given the immeasurable number of comorbidities that individuals with autism can be expected to experience, it is imperative that substance misuse workers have a working understanding of the varying social issues potentially impacting this group.

While the use of substances has significantly negative impacts on the life of an individual with an Autism Spectrum Condition (ASC), the impacts of substance misuse are compounded. Substance misuse impacts physical health, mental health, and social and occupational functioning. Substance misuse can also make co-occurring physical health complaints worse, possibly having a direct effect on contemporary life. Additionally, individuals with autism are observed to have a higher rate of physical health complaints, meaning they would potentially benefit far more from the support of a drug worker than a non-autistic individual might. Autism can affect behavioral and cognitive responses, which has implications for substance use and misuse. Moreover, individuals may be excluded from substance misuse treatment services due to either an assumption of vulnerability based on the existence of an ASC, or of their autism excluding them from the service entirely. These ultimately risk the lives of these individuals.

7.1. Physical Health

In conclusion, for those with physical health problems, there is a general lack of research looking at these in forensic populations, making it challenging to review the health of people in detention and who misuse substances. The implications for clinical practice from the relatively few studies that were identified include the importance of effective screening for tuberculosis and closer supervision of those with HCV undergoing surgical treatment. When working with people with ASD in relation to their substance use, physical well-being seems to be overlooked. If one-fifth, or more, of people with Asperger's syndrome have a co-morbid mental health disorder, such as depression, this could be considered a significant clinical issue if not assessed alongside co-morbid substance misuse. Combining the results from this systemic review with the additional published literature, there is a pressing need to address the physical health of adults with ASD if we are able to have substance misuse interventions that are truly holistic.

Misuse of substances: Whilst it is beyond the scope of this review to consider how symptoms of ASD may contribute to or protect against substance misuse, there are substantial concerns about the physical health implications of substance misuse for people with ASD. Adults with substance use disorders are significantly more likely than individuals without such disorders to experience a variety of physical health problems, including respiratory and circulatory problems, gastrointestinal difficulties, arthritis, hepatitis, tuberculosis, cancer, and sexually transmitted diseases. Drug misusers have rates of hepatitis C, for example, 50 times the national average. Mental health problems and suicidal ideation are also higher than in the rest of the general population. In addition to the risk of dependence, the National Institute of Clinical Excellence has reported that people with ASD, who tend to prefer routine and have difficulty adapting to new environments, may be more vulnerable to addiction than the general population and may find it harder to give up addictive substances. With regards to people who misuse drugs requiring surgical care, it is reported that post-operative sepsis was relatively common as well as gross behavioral problems at the time of admission. Lastly, substance misuse treatment can be more challenging when someone has a mental health problem and/or a learning disability. There is concern, therefore, that dealing effectively with substance misuse might be restricted to focusing solely on the mental health of an individual with ASD who misuses drugs; interventions for substance misuse that include physical health care will not necessarily intervene appropriately with individuals who have normal intellectual functioning alongside ASD.

7.2. Mental Health

In summary, it is clear that in addition to the risks to physical health, substance misuse can have a significant and negative impact on the mental health of individuals with autism. As such, an integrated approach is required in the provision of services to address substance misuse problems, mental health issues, and comorbidities for all people, including individuals with autism, who misuse substances. Specific training will enhance the skills and knowledge of staff working in drug treatment services, including: increasing the understanding of autism and associated challenges; encouraging early identification, assessment, and referral to secondary substance misuse services for those with possible autism; providing guidance on effective assessment of people with autism and substance misuse; and giving tools and resources to support effective intervention and engagement of people with autism.

Substance misuse can exacerbate underlying mental health issues, with substance use-related difficulties also being strongly linked to worsening mental health. Almost 50% of prisoners report that they were under the influence of drugs or alcohol at the time of their offense, and one in three individuals attending A&E with an injury has alcohol in their system. For individuals with autism who also misuse substances, the impact on their mental health and behavior can be profound. In particular, there is evidence to suggest that alcohol and illicit drugs, such as cannabis, can worsen underlying mental health conditions, such as anxiety, mood, and eating disorders. There is also some evidence to suggest that the use of some substances can increase the occurrence of a number of the key symptoms of autism, such as problems with social behavior and communication, increases in anxiety and depression, obsessions and compulsions, and higher levels of aggression. However, research suggests that there is a lack of formal services available to address both the substance misuse and comorbid mental health issues of individuals with autism. What little anecdotal evidence there is suggests that people with autism who misuse substances feel that they are 'falling between the two stools' of addiction and mental health services.

7.3. Social and Occupational Functioning

The social and relationship context is one where much less is known. With the often-touted social impairments characteristic of autism spectrum disorder (ASD), social isolation and potential substance use may be an even greater area of risk. For example, friendships formed around substance use are associated with more problematic patterns of use in non-autistic community samples and could potentially lead to more serious impairment in the daily lives of those on the autistic spectrum. Problematic substance use may also contribute to unemployment or trouble holding jobs, as has been noted in the very limited literature that touches on issues of work and employment in people on the autistic spectrum. It is thus possible that substance misuse can impact on the stressful pattern of social exclusion and unemployment that has been seen in people at high functioning ends of the autism spectrum and exacerbate the functional problems associated with the disorder of employment and social functioning. These negative secondary social outcomes, rather than direct effects of substance use, are likely to require a multi-disciplinary approach encompassing the social, psychological, physical, and clinical domains.

7.3. Social and Occupational Functioning, daily life and social participation. Substance misuse is associated with increased risk of social isolation, impairments in social relationships, family breakdown, and homelessness. The level of functional impairment directly corresponds to the frequency of substance use, and individuals with more severe substance dependence tend to have less stable accommodation and employment. Alcohol and drug use are also linked to prolonged periods of unemployment, reduced progression in education, and fewer years of formal education. Drug and alcohol use can also contribute to associated co-occurring issues, such as criminal offending, that can further disrupt social relationships and result in social exclusion.

8. Interventions and Treatment Strategies

Interventions include behavioral therapies, pharmacological interventions, family supports including group interventions and "even a helpful service dog who is part of a treatment protocol as one lowers dosage of psychiatric medications," and other supportive community programs. Some consideration is given to developmental processes and an individual's previous history of overcoming challenges in the selection of treatment. The impulsive tendencies that sometimes lead someone to end a course of treatment against medical advice could be ameliorated with longer-term incentive/motivational interventions. For the autistic community, a similar array of strategies might be considered, to address the complexities that may underlie a substance use issue.

In order to support those who are affected by both autism and substance use challenges, a variety of interventions are designed to equip them with necessary skills and resources to effectively cope with difficulties. The Collaborative Interventions for Circles of Support project developed a family psychoeducation group (FPG) treatment. Family psychoeducation is based on evidence that suggests that keeping families informed and involved in therapy can improve long-term treatment outcome for a variety of psychiatric diagnoses. Currently, practicality and effectiveness of this form of treatment still need to be evaluated for co-occurring autism and substance use challenges. Interventions for those with substance use issues generally involve a multi-pronged approach to promoting support, treatment, and rehabilitation. It is suggested that early intervention and treatment "in specialized and integrated care services improves substance abuse prognosis."

8.1. Behavioral Therapies

Behavioral therapies have historical and theoretical grounding in various principles of learning and behavior change. These principles can be applied in a variety of treatment approaches to effectively address the challenges of the ASD/ID population. In general, behavioral therapies focus on the relationship between behavior and the environment and on behavioral influences, including antecedents and consequences that maintain a behavior. Techniques include positive reinforcement and prompts, environmental modifications (e.g., reducing environmental stressors), functional behavioral assessment and functional behavior analysis, operant behavioral principles, social learning theory principles, and token economies. Group treatment approaches, including those using peer-mediated strategies (e.g., peer modeling), function on the same theoretical framework as individual treatments. In individuals with ASD, behavioral therapies address specific challenges and abilities. For example, social skills training and relationship skills training address challenges in social relationships in those with ASD. The type of intervention selected and the delivery are contingent upon the individual's skills, strengths, and deficits. The goals include the promotion of behaviors, enhancement of positive or adaptive behavioral repertoires, and reduction of undesirable behaviors. Any or all of these techniques can be behaviorally modified such that treatment of SUD in persons with ASD incorporates the treatment of ASD. In addition, specific behavioral therapies also have unique features that lend themselves to better adaptation/modification to persons with ASD and/or intellectual disability (ID).

SUDs occur in some individuals with autism with varying degrees of severity, suggesting the potential requirement of specialized interventions for this population. However, evidence for interventions for SUD in those with ASD often lacks efficacy. Although psychopharmacologic agents can be helpful in addressing multiple symptom domains in ASD, the relative efficacy of these agents for individuals with both SUD and ASD is greatly unknown. In the absence of controlled research, careful clinical management and moral individualized decision making is the best guideline for psychopharmacology selection and medication management. It is of great importance to begin to have some experimental data to begin drawing evidence-based treatment recommendations. The possibility of substance misuse underscores the importance of developing skills, strategies, and interventions in those with ASD to mitigate both the risk of the development of SUD and also treatment interventions for those with SUD.

8.2. Pharmacological Interventions

Medications should be used alongside existing evidence-based psychosocial treatments, such as relapse prevention, cognitive-behavioral therapy, and 12-step programs. As the role of medications is in an initial phase for autistic individuals, this report does not contain a specific intervention recommendation. Rather, the working group identified the need for a comprehensive approach in managing substance misuse, which included psychological and social input. Medications should therefore be seen as a complementary addition to evidence-based psychosocial approaches, tailored to the individual if they have been helpful historically.

A number of medications have been trialled for treating substance misuse and are available for clinicians to use. Antidepressants, in particular selective serotonin reuptake inhibitors (SSRIs) and tricyclic antidepressants, are commonly used due to their potential to reduce symptoms of anxiety, which often co-occur with substance misuse. Although a large body of evidence has shown SSRIs' efficacy in reducing alcohol dependence, there is less evidence to support the use of medications to treat illicit substance misuse. The only other medication pathway for which there is solid evidence at present is oral naltrexone for opiate dependence. Naltrexone is an opioid receptor antagonist and is thought to work by keeping an individual off opioids (predominantly heroin) by reducing the pleasurable effects. As support with substance misuse is essential at the same time, the development of oral naltrexone could be seen as a useful adjunct in breaking the cycle of substance misuse. A number of other medications are also under investigation at present for treating smoking, cannabis, and cocaine misuse.

8.3. Family and Community Support Programs

Sally has asserted that the resilience and sensitivity of the population that goes on to be defined as autistic to substances and drugs, however, are high enough for substance use to contribute to and increase autism-specific illnesses, including self-harm, burn-out, and malware. The Scottish Women's Autism Network (SWAN) research in 2016 of 35 Scottish women over 35 with a formal diagnosis of autism highlighted their struggles to avoid drugs of all kinds. This research was also backed up by the work of a group of autistic adults researching the 'Skills for learning, life and work' Curriculum for Excellence users, which also highlighted the use of drugs and alcohol across the autism population. Furthermore, programs of advocacy and social and emotional mentoring within schools have presented concerns from primary school children and parents. It is clear that rather than hiding drugs and alcohol being used, a collective societal response across community programs that includes addressing drugs will be necessary to start a conversation about positive engagement with drugs.

Family and community-based support was identified as a positive resource in the research into substance misuse. To be valued and pursued, it needs to be understood as materially and quantitatively diffused in society. Research into relevant services suggests a balance of needs and outcomes across the autistic population, including struggling with or avoiding drugs and alcohol. This includes those who have chosen to abstain altogether and those who have fought a battle to be an occasional social drinker. If the potential outcomes of drinking or drug misuse are seen as autism and/or mental health specific, then it is easier to address people's fears and start a dialogue about moving forward.

9. Future Directions in Research and Practice

Overall, this short review reveals a complex field of risk factors for substance misuse in autistic people. It also highlights the current gulf in practice and knowledge in how to support autistic people with substance misuse difficulties. The development of pathways is a much-needed first step. Further research into the phenomenological similarities and differences observed in 'self-medication' and 'interactional' substance misuse are also recommended, in order to further develop specific pathways and hypothetical tailored to the particular need of each group. As research in this field progresses, it is likely that more evidence-based prevention resources will become available, and theoretical considerations on strategies for substance misuse will become more sophisticated.

The preceding sections of this essay have discussed the different factors in current evidence that are associated with substance misuse by autistic people. Clearly, there is a strong need for more work on prevention, diagnosis, assessment, and care for autistic people with complex needs. A vast area of research is currently untapped. The responses can be very different regarding genetic, environmental, and developmental backgrounds, as well as individual attributes, family resources, and societal opportunities. Work is urgently needed on the interactions between mental health difficulties alongside neurodevelopmental conditions, social disadvantage, school exclusions, and other vulnerability factors. This may pave the way for advances in developing interventions to bring about improved quality of life and social inclusion and to enable responsible transitions to adult services. This suggests that initial work should focus on broadening pathways for children and young people seeking help regarding substance misuse.

www.ingramcontent.com/pod-product-compliance
Lightning Source LLC
Chambersburg PA
CBHW050832260726

48660CB00006B/2198